FOGSI EEBR 2025

Ethical Evidence-Based Recommendations

Hyperglycemia in Pregnancy

Disclaimer

This Ethical Evidence-Based Recommendation (EEBR) document is drafted following a consensus between esteemed FOGSI experts and stakeholders and are based on the scientific evidence available at the time of preparation.

EEBRs should be used for information and educational purposes. They do not replace the need for application of clinical judgment to each individual presentation, or variations based on individual patient and resource setting.

Furthermore, EEBRs do not constitute or imply the endorsement of any of the included technologies, therapies, or techniques by FOGSI.

FOGSI EEBR 2025

Ethical Evidence-Based Recommendations

Hyperglycemia in Pregnancy

Editor-in-Chief

Sunita Tandulwadkar
MD (Obs and Gyne) FICS (Gyne-Endoscopy) FICOG
President, FOGSI (2025–2026)
Gynecological Endoscopist and ART & IVF Specialist
Head, Department of Obstetrics and Gynecology
Chief, IVF & Endoscopy Center, Ruby Hall Clinic, Pune
Founder and Medical Director
Solo Clinic IVF—A Center for Excellence in Infertility and Endoscopy, Pune
Founder and Medical Director
Solo Stem Cells—A Stem Cell Research and Application Center, Pune
Founder and Director, Alive Regenerative Wellness, Pune, Maharashtra, India

Editor

Charmila Ayyavoo
MD DGO DFP FICOG PGDCR
Director and Consultant
Department of Obstetrics and Gynecology
Aditi Hospital, Tiruchirappalli
Dhanalakshmi Srinivasan Medical College
Tiruchirappalli, Tamil Nadu, India

Experts

Hema Divakar MD FRCOG
Senior Consultant and
Medical Director
Department of Obstetrics and
Gynecology
Divakars Speciality Hospital
Bengaluru, Karnataka, India

Parag Biniwale MD FICOG
Chief Consultant and Director
Department of Obstetrics and Gynecology
Biniwale Clinic
Pune, Maharashtra, India
Chairman, ICOG 2025
Past President
Pune Obstetric and Gynaecological Society

Convener

Pooja Lodha DNB (Obs and Gyne)
Fellow, Fetal Medicine, FOGSI-FMF UK Certified
Lead Consultant
Department of Fetal Medicine
Ruby Hall Clinic and Bharati Vidyapeeth University and Hospital, Pune
Director, Kangaroo Cradle, Fetal Care Centre
Pune, Maharashtra, India

JAYPEE BROTHERS MEDICAL PUBLISHERS
The Health Sciences Publisher
New Delhi | London

Jaypee Brothers Medical Publishers (P) Ltd

Headquarters
Jaypee Brothers Medical Publishers (P) Ltd
EMCA House, 23/23-B
Ansari Road, Daryaganj
New Delhi 110 002, India
Landline: +91-11-23272143, +91-11-23272703
+91-11-23282021, +91-11-23245672
Email: jaypee@jaypeebrothers.com

Corporate Office
Jaypee Brothers Medical Publishers (P) Ltd
4838/24, Ansari Road, Daryaganj
New Delhi 110 002, India
Phone: +91-11-43574357
Fax: +91-11-43574314
Email: jaypee@jaypeebrothers.com

Overseas Office
JP Medical Ltd.
83, Victoria Street, London
SW1H 0HW (UK)
Phone: +44 20 3170 8910
Fax: +44 (0)20 3008 6180
Email: info@jpmedpub.com

Website: www.jaypeebrothers.com
Website: www.jaypeedigital.com

Inquiries for bulk sales may be solicited at: jaypee@jaypeebrothers.com

FOGSI EEBR 2025—Ethical Evidence-Based Recommendations: Hyperglycemia in Pregnancy

First Edition: **2025**

ISBN: 978-93-6616-731-2

Printed in India

Contributors

AG Radhika
MBBS DGO DNB MNAMS FICOG
Senior Consultant
Department of Obstetrics and Gynecology
Guru Teg Bahadur Hospital
New Delhi, India

Ahila Ayyavoo
DCH DNB (Pediatrics) Fellowship in Pediatric Endocrinology (NZ) PhD (NZ)
Consultant, Pediatric Endocrinology and Diabetes
Department of Pediatrics
G Kuppuswamy Naidu Memorial Hospital and
Masonic Medical Centre for Children
Coimbatore, Tamil Nadu, India

Archana Chaudhary MBBS MS
Specialist Grade 1
Department of Obstetrics and Gynecology
Guru Teg Bahadur Hospital
New Delhi, India

Bhavatharini Aruyerchelvan
MBBS D Diabetology
Senior Consultant Diabetologist
Department of Diabetes
SRC Diabetes Care Center
Erode, Tamil Nadu, India

Charmila Ayyavoo
MD DGO DFP FICOG PGDCR
Director and Consultant
Department of Obstetrics and Gynecology
Aditi Hospital, Tiruchirappalli
Dhanalakshmi Srinivasan Medical College
Tiruchirappalli, Tamil Nadu, India

Hema Divakar MD FRCOG
Senior Consultant and Medical Director
Department of Obstetrics and Gynecology
Divakars Speciality Hospital
Bengaluru, Karnataka, India

Meeta Gupta
MS MBBS FICOG FIMSA MAMS ACME
Professor and Head
Department of Obstetrics and Gynecology
All India Institute of Medical Sciences
Jammu, Jammu and Kashmir, India

Parag Biniwale MD FICOG
Chief Consultant and Director
Department of Obstetrics and Gynecology
Biniwale Clinic
Pune, Maharashtra, India
Chairman, ICOG 2025
Past President, Pune Obstetric and Gynaecological Society

R Aruyerchelvan MD D Diabetology
Senior Consultant
Department of Diabetology
SRC Diabetes Care Center
Erode, Tamil Nadu, India

S Karthikeyan
MBBS DCH DNB (Pediatrics) FIPP AASC FAAP
Assistant Professor and Consultant
Department of Pediatrics and Pediatric Pulmonology
KAPV Government Medical College
Aditi Hospital, Maa Kauvery,
KMC Speciality Hospital
Tiruchirappalli, Tamil Nadu, India

Sujata Misra MD FICOG
Director
Department of Obstetrics and Gynecology
Postgraduate Institute of Medical Education and Research and Capital Hospital
Bhubaneswar, Odisha, India

Sunita Tandulwadkar
MD (Obs and Gyne) FICS (Gyne-Endoscopy) FICOG
President, FOGSI (2025–2026)
Gynecological Endoscopist and ART & IVF Specialist
Head, Department of Obstetrics and Gynecology
Chief, IVF & Endoscopy Center
Ruby Hall Clinic, Pune
Founder and Medical Director
Solo Clinic IVF—A Center for Excellence in Infertility and Endoscopy, Pune
Founder and Medical Director
Solo Stem Cells—A Stem Cell Research and Application Center, Pune
Founder and Director
Alive Regenerative Wellness
Pune, Maharashtra, India

Uma Ram DGO DNB FRCOG
Director and OBGYN Lead
Department of Obstetrics and Gynecology
Seethapathy Clinic and Hospital
Chennai, Tamil Nadu, India

Veerasamy Seshiah
MD FRCP FACP DSc (Hony)
Honorary Distinguished Professor
Department of Diabetology
The Tamil Nadu Dr MGR Medical University
Chennai, Tamil Nadu, India

Preface

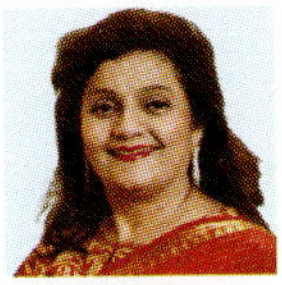

Editor-in-Chief
Sunita Tandulwadkar

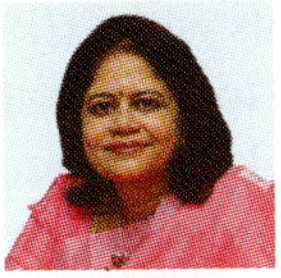

Editor
Charmila Ayyavoo

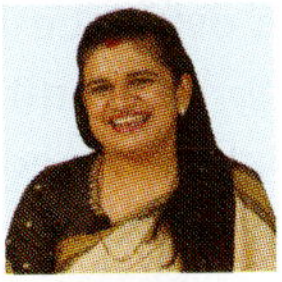

Expert
Hema Divakar

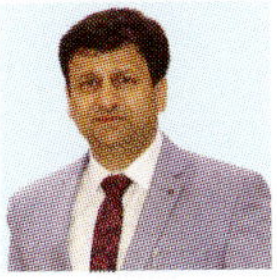

Expert
Parag Biniwale

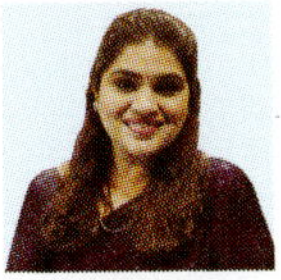

Convener
Pooja Lodha

In our quest to improve maternal and neonatal outcomes in India, it is crucial that we build a foundation of ethical evidence-based guidelines for managing complex conditions. As the President of the Federation of Obstetric and Gynaecological Societies of India (FOGSI) 2025, I am honored to introduce this comprehensive guide on *Hyperglycemia in Pregnancy*, a key resource for obstetricians in providing informed, effective care to pregnant individuals facing this prevalent challenge. While international bodies such as International Federation of Gynecology and Obstetrics (FIGO), American Society for Reproductive Medicine (ASRM), and Royal College of Obstetricians and Gynaecologists (RCOG) have developed guidelines addressing hyperglycemia in pregnancy (HIP), this book marks India's step toward creating a specialized and locally relevant resource. Our aim is to bridge existing gaps, giving Indian practitioners a reliable guide for managing HIP, adapted to the specific needs of our patients and healthcare system.

This book addresses all aspects of HIP, beginning with essential definitions, classification, and epidemiology. These foundational chapters set the stage by clarifying the scope and significance of HIP, providing practitioners with a clear understanding of its prevalence and implications for maternal and fetal health. Recognizing the importance of proactive management, we delve into preconceptional optimization, an often-overlooked but vital step to ensure healthier pregnancies by stabilizing blood glucose levels even before conception.

Guidance on gestational diabetes mellitus (GDM) screening and diagnosis follows, offering evidence-based approaches to identifying gestational diabetes early and accurately. The medical management chapters provide insights into tailored treatment strategies for both gestational diabetes and preexisting diabetes (type 1 and type 2) during pregnancy, considering the unique physiological demands of each case.

Moving into obstetric management, this book outlines recommendations for safely managing pregnancy and labor in the context of HIP, detailing monitoring practices and interventions designed to protect both maternal and neonatal health. Further, the neonatal management chapter provides protocols for immediate and effective care of newborns affected by maternal hyperglycemia, addressing key concerns such as hypoglycemia and respiratory issues.

The book also includes guidance on both short-term and long-term care, recognizing that HIP requires ongoing attention beyond delivery. This includes recommendations on postpartum follow-up and lifestyle modifications to reduce future risks for both mother and child. Additionally, a dedicated chapter on contraceptive choices for individuals with HIP helps practitioners to offer safe family planning advice tailored to each patient's needs, while the final chapter examines the potential complications associated with HIP, preparing obstetricians to anticipate and manage these risks effectively.

We hope that this book serves as a valuable tool for healthcare providers across India, supporting them in delivering compassionate, evidence-based care for those impacted by hyperglycemia in pregnancy. This initiative represents FOGSI's commitment to advancing maternal and neonatal health and empowering practitioners with the knowledge they need to make informed and patient-centered decisions.

Contents

CHAPTER 1

Definition, Classification, and Epidemiology of Hyperglycemia in Pregnancy

Meeta Gupta

Q1. What is the definition of HIP?

Hyperglycemia in pregnancy refers to elevated blood glucose (sugar) levels during pregnancy.

It typically occurs in two forms:

1. *Gestational diabetes mellitus (GDM):* This is the most common form of hyperglycemia during pregnancy. It develops during pregnancy, and usually resolves after childbirth. GDM can increase the risk of complications for both the mother and the baby, including pre-eclampsia, preterm birth, and increased birth weight.
2. *Preexisting diabetes:* Some women may have pre-existing Type 1 or Type 2 diabetes before becoming pregnant. This condition requires careful management throughout the pregnancy to avoid complications.

Q2. What are the diagnostic criteria as per different guidelines?

The diagnostic criteria for Hyperglycemia in Pregnancy (HIP) vary depending on the guidelines used. The most referenced guidelines are from the International Association of Diabetes and Pregnancy Study Groups (IADPSG), the World Health Organization (WHO), and the American Diabetes Association (ADA).

The Government of India recognizes the Diabetes in Pregnancy Study Group India *(DIPSI)* Criteria. It is as follows:

- *When:* During the first antenatal visit and/or at 24–28 weeks.
- *Test:* 75 g OGTT, nonfasting. (irrespective of last meal)
- *Diagnostic criteria:* 2-hour postglucose load ≥140 mg/dL (7.8 mmol/L)
- *Diagnosis:* GDM is diagnosed if this value is met or exceeded.

Q3. What is the global and Indian prevalence of hyperglycemia of pregnancy?

Hyperglycemia is considered a silent global epidemic.

WHO estimates that 16.9% of pregnancies globally are affected by hyperglycemia in pregnancy contributing to 21.4 million of 127.1 million live births.

The International Diabetes Federation (IDF) estimated in 2019 (9th edition) the global prevalence of diabetes in pregnancy was 15.5% with 12.8% GDM, 1.3% preexisting diabetes 1.3%, and 1.3% as diabetes first detected in pregnancy. Southeast Asia has the highest prevalence of GDM with an estimated prevalence of 23–25%, contributing to 6.9 million live births with India, being the largest populous country and diabetic capital of the world showing the prevalence of GDM ranging from about 3 to 35%.

Q4. How do socioeconomic status, ethnicity, and geographic location influence the epidemiology of hyperglycemia of pregnancy?

Socioeconomic status especially lifestyle changes like rapid urbanization, dietary shifts toward high-calorie, processed foods, obesity and decreased physical activity have significantly contributed to this rising prevalence of HIP.

- *Geographic location:* Urban Areas have higher prevalence, often exceeding 25%, due to lifestyle factors, higher rates of obesity, and a more sedentary lifestyle.
- *Rural areas:* Slightly lower prevalence, but it is rising due to changes in diet and physical activity levels.
- *Southern India:* Studies have reported some of the highest prevalence rates, ranging from 17% to 35%.
- *Northern and Eastern India:* Slightly lower rates, around 10–20%, but these are still significant.

"Among 803 164 sampled individuals [691,982 (86.2%) women; mean (SD) age, 30.09 (9.97) years], substantial geographic variation in diabetes prevalence in India was found, with a concentrated burden at the southern coastline [cluster 1, Andhra Pradesh and Telangana: prevalence, 3.01% (1864 of 61,948 individuals); cluster 2, Tamil Nadu and Kerala: prevalence, 4.32% (3,429 of 79,435 individuals); cluster 3, east Orissa: prevalence, 2.81% (330 of 11,758 individuals); cluster 4, Goa: prevalence, 4.43% (83 of individuals)].

Ethnicity: Genetic Predisposition in South Asians including Indians has a higher genetic susceptibility to insulin resistance, contributing to higher rates of GDM.

Q5. What trends have been observed in the epidemiology of hyperglycemia of pregnancy over the past few decades?

The epidemiology of hyperglycemia in pregnancy has seen significant changes over the past few decades, with a notable increase in prevalence driven by factors such as rising obesity rates, older maternal age, and improved screening practices.

These trends highlights are due to factors like:

- *Rising prevalence:*
    - *Global increase:* The prevalence of hyperglycemia in pregnancy has been steadily increasing across the globe. This rise is largely attributed to the growing obesity epidemic, changes in diet, and reduced physical activity.

- *Developing countries:* The increase is particularly pronounced in low- and middle-income countries, where rapid urbanization and lifestyle shifts have contributed to a surge in GDM cases.
- *High-income countries:* In developed countries, the prevalence of GDM has also risen, partly due to more widespread and rigorous screening programs and the trend toward later childbearing.

- *Shift toward older maternal age:*
  - *Delayed childbearing:* There has been a trend toward women having children at older ages, a demographic shift that is associated with an increased risk of GDM. Advanced maternal age is a significant risk factor due to increased insulin resistance.
  - *Impact on GDM rates:* As more women delay pregnancy into their 30s and 40s, the incidence of hyperglycemia in pregnancy has risen accordingly.
- *Impact of obesity and lifestyle factors:*
  - *Obesity epidemic:* The global rise in obesity is one of the strongest drivers of the increasing prevalence of GDM. Obesity is closely linked to insulin resistance, which is a major factor in the development of GDM.
  - *Sedentary lifestyles:* The global shift toward more sedentary lifestyles, especially in urban areas, has contributed to higher rates of GDM.
  - *Dietary changes:* The widespread adoption of diets high in refined sugars and unhealthy fats has exacerbated the risk of GDM, particularly in populations transitioning from traditional to more Westernized diets.
- *Enhanced screening and diagnosis:*
  - *Wider screening programs:* Increased awareness and better healthcare infrastructure have led to the implementation of more widespread screening for GDM, particularly in countries where it was previously underdiagnosed.
  - *Refined diagnostic criteria:* The adoption of standardized and more sensitive diagnostic criteria, such as those from the International Association of Diabetes and Pregnancy Study Groups (IADPSG), has contributed to a rise in diagnosed cases.
- *Ethnic and geographical variations:*
  - *Regional differences:* The prevalence of GDM varies widely by region, with higher rates observed in Southeast Asia, the Middle East, and certain parts of Africa and Latin America. These differences are influenced by genetic, environmental, and socioeconomic factors.
  - *Ethnic disparities:* Certain ethnic groups, including South Asians, Hispanic Americans, African Americans, and Indigenous populations, have higher rates of GDM compared to other groups, reflecting genetic predispositions and lifestyle factors.

- *Socioeconomic influences:*
  - *Impact of socioeconomic status:* Socioeconomic factors, such as income and education, play a significant role in the prevalence and management of GDM. Lower socioeconomic status is often associated with higher GDM rates due to limited access to healthcare, poor nutrition, and lack of awareness.
  - *Urbanization:* The shift from rural to urban living has been linked to an increase in GDM, as urban environments often promote less physical activity and more calorie-dense diets.

Q6. How have changes in diagnostic criteria influenced the reported prevalence of hyperglycemia of pregnancy?

Changes in diagnostic criteria for hyperglycemia in pregnancy, particularly the shift to more inclusive and sensitive thresholds, have led to an increase in the reported prevalence of the condition. The adoption of lower glucose thresholds, universal screening practices, and the transition to one-step testing methods have all contributed to a higher detection rate of GDM, reflecting a more comprehensive understanding and recognition of the condition's impact on maternal and fetal health.

- *Broader and more inclusive criteria due to lower thresholds and one abnormal value versus two values:* These lower thresholds mean that more women are now classified as having GDM compared to older criteria, which had higher cutoff values. Older criteria often required two abnormal values for a diagnosis. This shift has significantly increased the number of women diagnosed with GDM.
- *Adoption of universal screening and timing and frequency of the screening:* Universal screening captures more cases, including those in women who might not have been tested under selective screening protocols, thus increasing the reported prevalence. Early screening also identifies women with undiagnosed preexisting diabetes or early-onset GDM, adding to the prevalence figures.
- *Differences between one-step and two-step approaches:* The two-step approach generally results in a lower prevalence compared to the one-step method, but as more regions adopt the one-step approach, the reported prevalence has risen.
- *Increased sensitivity of tests due to improved detection and enhanced laboratory standards:* More sensitive and standardized tests have been developed, improving the accuracy of GDM diagnosis. These advancements and better laboratory standards have reduced the number of missed cases and increased the overall detection rate leading to an apparent increase in GDM prevalence.

Q7. What is the paternal influence of hyperglycemia in offspring?

The children of diabetic fathers can develop diabetes by direct epigenetic and genetic influences as well as indirect influences. Paternal age and environmental exposures can also alter the transmission to the offspring. The nongenetic paternal influence is through the postnatal environment. The father's eating habits, cultural and social influences can affect the offspring's lifestyle.

Q8. What are the current research gaps in the study of hyperglycemia of pregnancy, and what future directions might research take?

The study of hyperglycemia in pregnancy, including gestational diabetes mellitus (GDM) and preexisting diabetes, has advanced significantly, but several research gaps are remaining. Here are some key research gaps and potential future directions:

- *Pathophysiology and mechanisms:* The role of the placenta in modulating glucose metabolism and the interaction between maternal, fetal, and placental factors require more detailed study.
- *Individualized risk prediction:* Current screening methods for GDM are largely population-based and do not account for individual variability in risk. There is a need for better risk stratification to identify women who would benefit most from early intervention.
- *Long-term outcomes for mothers and offspring:* The long-term effects of different GDM management strategies on the risk of developing type 2 diabetes mellitus and cardiovascular disease in mothers and metabolic disorders in offspring are less clear.
- *Optimal screening and diagnostic criteria:* The adoption of different criteria (e.g., IADPSG vs. ADA vs. DIPSI) leads to variability in diagnosis and management. The cost-effectiveness and clinical outcomes of different screening strategies are not fully understood.
- *Impact of lifestyle interventions:* While lifestyle interventions, including diet and physical activity, are known to reduce GDM risk, the specific types, intensities, and timing of these interventions that are most effective remain unclear.
- *Management of hyperglycemia in pregnancy:* The long-term effects of different management strategies on both mothers and children are not well understood.
- *Psychosocial and behavioral aspects:* The psychosocial impact of a GDM diagnosis on pregnant women, including stress, anxiety, and adherence to treatment, is not fully understood.
- *Global and regional disparities:* There are significant disparities in the prevalence, diagnosis, and management of GDM across different regions and populations. Understanding the factors contributing to these

disparities, including genetic, environmental, and healthcare access issues, is critical.

- *Implications of GDM on future generations:* The concept of "fetal programming," where in utero exposure to hyperglycemia may predispose offspring to metabolic diseases, requires further investigation.
- *Integration of technology in GDM management:* The effectiveness, acceptability, and cost-effectiveness of technologies like continuous glucose monitoring (CGM) and telemedicine, in GDM management need further study.

Addressing these research gaps will require a multidisciplinary approach, integrating insights from genetics, endocrinology, public health, psychology, and technology. By focusing on these areas, future research can improve the understanding, prevention, and management of hyperglycemia in pregnancy, ultimately reducing its impact on maternal and child health. Addressing these gaps will also improve our understanding, prevention strategies and management of hyperglycemia in pregnancy, ultimately enhancing maternal and fetal health outcomes.

BIBLIOGRAPHY

1. Hernandez AM, Jia P, Kim HY, et al. Geographic variation and associated covariates of diabetes prevalence in India. JAMA Netw Open. 2020;3(5):e203865. Erratum in: JAMA Netw Open. 20201;3(5):e2010311.
2. McCance D. Diabetes in Pregnancy. Best Pract Res Clin Obstet Gynaecol. 2015;29:685-99.
3. Nanditha A, Ma RC, Ramachandran A, et al. Diabetes in Asia and the Pacific: Implications for the Global Epidemic. Diabetes Care. 2016;39:472-85.
4. Penesova A, Bunt JC, Bogardus C, et al. Effect of paternal diabetes on pre-diabetic phenotypes in adult offspring. Diabetes Care. 2010;33(8):1823-8.
5. Seshiah V, Balaji V, Balaji MS, et al. Gestational diabetes mellitus in India. J Assoc Physicians India. 2004;52:707-11.
6. Yuen L, Saeedia P, Riaz M, et al. Projections of the prevalence of hyperglycaemia in pregnancy in 2019 and beyond: Results from the International Diabetes Federation Diabetes Atlas, 9th Diabetes Research and Clinical Practice. 2019;157:1-12.

CHAPTER 2

Preconceptional Optimization

Charmila Ayyavoo

Q1. What are the risk factors for developing GDM?

Draft recommendation: Overweight women, past delivery of a baby with macrosomia, history of GDM in previous pregnancies, history of diabetes in a first degree relative, older maternal age, South Asian population, physical inactivity, hypertension, Low levels of HDL cholesterol, increased fasting triglycerides, history of Polycystic ovarian syndrome (PCOS), evidence of insulin resistance like acanthosis nigricans, morbid obesity, history of cardiovascular disease, history of HIV are risk factors for developing GDM.

Summary of evidence: The NICE Guidelines and ACOG guidelines have accepted that overweight women, past delivery of a baby with macrosomia, history of GDM in previous pregnancies, history of diabetes in a first degree relative, older maternal age, South Asian population are at increased risk of developing GDM. The ACOG guidelines describes additional risk factors like physical inactivity, hypertension, less levels of HDL cholesterol, increased fasting triglycerides, history of Polycystic ovarian syndrome (PCOS), evidence of insulin resistance like acanthosis nigricans, morbid obesity, history of cardiovascular disease and history of HIV.

Q2. What are the factors to be controlled in preconceptional period to reduce the chances of GDM?

Draft recommendation: Dietary patterns, body weight, exercise regime should be controlled in the preconceptional period.

Summary of evidence: Diet and physical activity in the pre-conceptional period, (risk difference – 0.03, 95% CI: 0.06, – 0.01; I^2: 58.69%), intake of inositol (risk difference – 0.19, 95% CI: 0.33, – 0.06; I^2: 92.19%), and use vitamin D helped to control GDM in mothers in a study by Quotah et al. (risk difference – 0.16, 95% CI: 0.25, – 0.06; I^2: 32.27%). In the analysis of subgroups in the in the study, diet and physical activity interventions were useful in women who had more than two risk factors for the development of GDM and inositol was found to be useful in women with obesity.

Q3. What is the lifestyle management in preconception?

Draft recommendation: A change in diet and exercise is made in the preconception period in women who have risk factors for developing GDM.

Summary of evidence: Diet and exercise in the preconceptional period can reduce the chance of a woman developing GDM according to a Cochrane review by Griffith et al. The review involved 19 trials and 6,633 women.

Q4. What are the targets for preconceptional blood glucose control in women with a history of GDM?

Draft recommendation: Fasting blood sugar levels <100 mg/dL and a 2-hour postprandial blood sugar level of 140 mg/dL.

Summary of evidence: GOI advises preconceptional testing of women with history of GDM. This will prevent the development of HIP with its attendant maternal and neonatal complications.

Q5. What are the targets of preconception control in type 1 diabetes in pregnancy?

Draft recommendation: Self-monitoring of blood sugars is mandatory in women who have diabetes before pregnancy. They should be taught about blood sugar targets in pregnancy and hypoglycemic attacks.

Summary of evidence: They should have a fasting blood sugar value of 90–126 mg/dL and 72–126 mg/dL before other meals. It is essential that the desired target levels of blood sugar be maintained in the preconceptional period to prevent congenital anomalies, spontaneous abortions, hypertension during pregnancy and other complications.

Q6. What is the role of glycosylated hemoglobin in the pre-conceptional period?

Draft recommendation: Women with diabetes planning pregnancy should maintain their HbA1c below 6.5%. This needs to be achieved without development of hypoglycemia.

Summary of evidence: The patients with type 1 diabetes should maintain the glycosylated hemoglobin below 6.5% to reduce maternal complications like hypertension and neonatal complications like macrosomia, hypoglycemia, shoulder dystocia, neonatal intensive care admissions. Along with medications, high glycemic carbohydrates intake should be reduced, and the weight gain of the mother should be controlled to maintain an optimum HbA1c.

Q7. What are the medications to be considered in the preconception?

Draft recommendation: Women with diabetes are advised to take tablet folic acid 5 mg from the preconception period till 12 weeks of gestation. Metformin, insulin therapy, are continued in the pre-conceptional period to maintain glycemic targets. Antihypertensive drugs which are safe in pregnancy are started in the preconceptional period after stopping the harmful drugs. Statins are discontinued in the preconceptional period.

Summary of evidence: Folic acid 5 mg is started in the pre-conceptional period to avoid neural tube defects in the fetus. Metformin is used as an alternative or as a combination with insulin therapy in the preconceptional period for an adequate control of blood sugar levels. Other oral hypoglycemic drugs are stopped as they are not as safe as metformin. Insulin therapy is needed in most of the diabetic patients for an adequate control. Regimes with newer insulins like aspart and lispro can be started in the preconceptional period. Long-acting insulins like Isophane insulin which is the regime of choice in pregnancy. Other long-acting insulin analogues like detemir or glargine are off-label even though they are safe during pregnancy.

Other medications: Antihypertensive drugs like angiotensin converting enzyme inhibitors and angiotensin II receptor antagonists are stopped once pregnancy is confirmed. Other anti-hypertensive drugs are started. Statins are stopped before or after pregnancy is confirmed.

Research gaps: Studies on the role of vitamin B12 in the development of HIP are needed. Research questions have been raised on the role of B12 deficiency in the development of insulin resistance and congenital anomalies.

Research has shown that excess levels of folate in first trimester are associated with hyperglycemia. The correct dose of periconceptional folic acid needs to be given with backing up of evidence.

Q8. How should the patient be counseled about fetal defects based on Glycosylated Hemoglobin?

Draft recommendation: If they maintain the HbA1c in the preconception period, the chances of congenital malformations in the baby are likely to be reduced. It is better not to conceive if the glycosylated hemoglobin levels are >10%.

Q9. What are the maternal assessments to be done in the preconceptional period?

Draft recommendation: A retinal and renal assessment are needed in women who have diabetes before pregnancy. For women with risk factors like obesity (BMI above 30 kg/m^2), a baby with macrosomia in an earlier pregnancy, history of gestational diabetes mellitus, history of diabetes in a first degree relative and ethnicity with a high risk of diabetes, screening for glucose intolerance can be done in the pre-conceptional period. For low-risk women, routine preconceptional care is enough.

Summary of evidence: A retinal and renal assessment are needed in a woman who has diabetes in the pre-conception period. A retinal assessment can be deferred if she had a retinal assessment in the last 6 months. Renal assessment in the form of measuring her urine albumin: creatinine ratio, serum creatinine and glomerular filtration rate (GFR) are done in the pre-conceptional period. She is referred to a nephrologist if her serum creatinine levels are more than 120 µmol/L; urine albumin: creatinine ratio is >30 mg/mL or the GFR is lesser than 45 mL/min/1.73 m^2.

BIBLIOGRAPHY

1. Benhalima K, Beunen K, Siegelaar SE, et al. Management of type 1 diabetes in pregnancy: update on lifestyle, pharmacological treatment, and novel technologies for achieving glycaemic targets. Lancet Diab Endocrinol. 2023;11(7):490-508.
2. Caughey AB, Turrentine M. ACOG Practice Bulletin: gestational diabetes mellitus. Obstet gynecol. 2018;131(2):E49-64.
3. Glinianaia SV, Tennant PWG, Bilous RW, et al. HbA1c and birthweight in women with pre-conception type 1 and type 2 diabetes: a population-based cohort study. Diabetologia. 2012; 55:3193-203.
4. Griffith RJ, Alsweiler J, Moore AE, et al. Interventions to prevent women from developing gestational diabetes mellitus: an overview of Cochrane reviews. Cochrane Database Syst Rev. 2020;6(6):CD012394.
5. NICE Guideline, 2015. Diabetes in pregnancy: management from preconception to the postnatal period. Guidance. London: National Institute for Health and Care Excellence (NICE); 2020.
6. Quotah OF, Andreeva D, Nowak KG, et al. Interventions in preconception and pregnant women at risk of gestational diabetes; a systematic review and meta-analysis of randomised controlled trials. Diabetol MetabolSyndr. 2024;16(1):8.

CHAPTER 3

Testing for Gestational Diabetes Mellitus

Charmila Ayyavoo

Q1. What is the target population for testing for gestational diabetes mellitus (GDM)?

Draft recommendation: All pregnant women at the first antenatal visit should undergo testing for GDM.

Summary of recommendation: Government of India (GOI), FIGO, DIPSI, and FOGSI advise that a universal screening for gestational diabetes mellitus be done for all pregnant women. There is a chance that GDM diagnosis will be missed if a selective screening is adopted rather than universal screening.

Q2. What is the protocol for testing?

Draft recommendation: The testing for GDM needs to be done two times during the antenatal period. The initial test is always done at the first antenatal visit of the mother. It is done as early as possible. If the first screening test is within normal limits, repeat testing is recommended between 24 and 28 weeks. If the first two screening tests are normal, repeat testing is recommended between 32–34 weeks.

Summary of evidence: The testing for GDM is based on the guidelines by GOI. If the first test is negative, the second test is done at 24–28 weeks of pregnancy. The second test is important as many women develop GDM at the end of the second trimester.

One third of patients with GDM are diagnosed in the first trimester. If a testing in the first trimester is missed, then it can be done at any time after 24 weeks of gestation. There needs to be a gap of 4 weeks between both the tests.

If the patient comes late in pregnancy for her first antenatal visit, it is imperative that a test for GDM is done at the instance of her first contact.

If she comes for her first antenatal visit only after 28 weeks of pregnancy, one test for GDM needs to be done.

If she tests positive for GDM at any test, management is as per protocol of Government of India Guidelines for GDM, 2018.

There is not necessary for the patient to be in fasting state as many pregnant women usually do not come in fasting state for antenatal checkups. Sampling of postglucose levels irrespective of meals is a simple and adequate test for GDM (Anjalakshi et al., 2009)

Q3. What is the test used for diagnosis?

Draft recommendation: It is a single step oral glucose challenge test.

Summary of evidence: The application of a single step test is based on GOI, FIGO, and DIPSI guidelines. The testing of fasting blood sugars and 2-hours postprandial blood sugars are advocated by FIGO guidelines for high resource settings. FIGO advocates testing for a single postprandial value in low resource settings which is also advised by DIPSI and GOI guidelines.

75 grams of glucose is dissolved in about 300 mL of water and the patient is asked to drink the glucose solution in 5–10 minutes. The patient can be fasting or nonfasting state. She should not leave the premises until the blood sugar testing is done after 2 hours. If she vomits within half an hour of the intake, the test is repeated the next day. If she has vomiting after half an hour of ingestion of glucose, the testing can be done on the same day.

The threshold for diagnosis is a blood sugar level of ≥140 mg/dL.

Q4. What is the instrument used for testing?

Draft recommendation: The plasma calibrated glucometer is used for getting the results at once. If a semi-auto-analyzer/auto-analyzer is available, they can be utilized for estimation of blood sugar values.

Summary of evidence: The instrument recommended for testing samples for GDM is based on GOI guidelines. It will be difficult to call pregnant patients to collect results on another day. They may miss coming. Hence, if centers do not have the expensive analyzer, the glucometer should be used to get results immediately and inform the patient on the same day.

It is necessary to have a glucometer in the labor room to monitor patients with GDM during labor.

The glucometer should be calibrated using calibration test strips or test solution as per the advice of the manufacturer.

BIBLIOGRAPHY

1. Anjalakshi C, Balaji V, Balaji MS, et al. A single test procedure to diagnose gestational diabetes mellitus. Acta Diabetol. 2009;46:51-4.
2. Cosson E, Benthimol M, Carbilon L. Universal screening for gestational diabetes mellitus improves maternal and fetal outcomes compared with selective screening. In: Mateclinsky FM (Ed). Abstract book of the 64th Scientific Sessions of the American Diabetes Association (ADA). Florida: American Diabetes Association; 2004. p. A61.
3. Endocrinology Committee FOGSI. Diagnosis and management of gestational diabetes mellitus guidelines by DIPSI (Revised) Vol 17, March 2021.
4. Hod M, Kapur A, Sacks DA, et al. The International Federation of Gynecology and Obstetrics (FIGO) Initiative on gestational diabetes mellitus: a pragmatic guide for diagnosis, management, and care. Int J Gynaecol Obstet. 2015;131(Suppl 3):S173-211.

5. Ministry of Health and Family welfare; Government of India. Diagnosis and management of gestational diabetes mellitus; Technical and Operational guidelines; Ministry of Health and Family welfare; Government of India; February 2018.
6. Neelakandan R, Sethu PS. Early universal screening for gestational diabetes mellitus. J Clin Diagn Res. 2014;8(4):OC12-4.
7. Seshiah V, Balaji V, Chawla R, et al. Diagnosis and management of gestational diabetes mellitus guidelines by DIPSI (Revised). Int J Diab Develop Countr. 2023;43(4):485-501.
8. Seshiah V, Shah SS, Balaji V, et al. When are we going to settle the diagnostic criteria of gestational diabetes mellitus. J Assoc Phys India. 2019;67:70-2.
9. Seshiah V. Clinical scoring in gestational diabetes screening. Int J Diabetes Dev Ctries. 2012;32:63-4.

CHAPTER 4

Management of Gestational Diabetes Mellitus

Sujata Misra

Q1. What are the guiding principles in the management of gestational diabetes mellitus (GDM)?

The guiding principles in the management of gestational diabetes mellitus (GDM) include:

- Lifestyle modifications in diet and exercise
- Insulin/oral hypoglycemic agents (OHA) wherever indicated
- Monitoring of blood glucose levels and maintaining an euglycemic status
- First trimester and second trimester screening for aneuploidy/anomalies
- Serial ultrasonic monitoring of fetal growth parameters
- Timely delivery and follow-up of the neonate.
- Postnatal follow-up for the glycemic status (ACOG)

Summary of evidence: FOGSI, ACOG, and the Government of India (GOI) have laid down guidelines for the management of GDM.

Q2. What are the dietary interventions and exercises advised in GDM?

Draft recommendation: Pregnant women diagnosed as GDM should be started on Medical Nutrition Therapy (MNT) and physical exercise for 2 weeks depending on the blood sugar levels.

After 2 weeks of MNT and physical exercise, if 2-hours PPBS is <120 mg/dL, the monitoring continues, and the test is repeated in every trimester. If 2-hours PPBS is ≥120 mg/dL insulin, or OHA should be initiated. Once diagnosed as a case of GDM, FBS, and 2-hours PPBS should be used to monitor the patient.

Summary of evidence: For the Indian population, GOI and FOGSI guidelines for dietary interventions and exercise are comprehensive.

Medical nutrition therapy (MNT): MNT refers to a carbohydrate controlled balanced meal plan which supports the nutritional requirement of the mother and the fetus. This is important for appropriate gestational weight gain and maintenance of normoglycemia.

The assessment includes defining her body mass index (BMI) and optimal pattern of weight gain during pregnancy. Calories and GDM Individualization are important when determining energy requirements and adjustments should be made accordingly.

Energy requirement does not increase in the first trimester unless a woman is underweight but increases in the second and third trimester.

As per Indian ICMR guidelines, an addition of 350 kcal/day above the adult requirement is recommended during second and third trimester for an average weight gain of 10–12 kg.

Severe caloric restriction should never be done as it may result in ketonemia and ketonuria and impair physical and mental development in offspring.

Based on the sugar levels and BMI of the patient, the nutritionist or physician should give them a personalized diet plan. The dietary recommendation should encompass caloric allotment and distribution and a proper balance of carbohydrate, protein, and fat intake.

Exercise: Regular 30 minutes of moderate-intensity aerobic exercise for at least 5 days a week is recommended. They should exercise for at least 50 minutes per week.

Q3. What is the "Gold standard" treatment in GDM?

Draft recommendation: If glycemic control is not achieved with diet and exercise, pharmacologic treatment is started. If the fasting blood glucose is >95 mg/dL or 1 hour glucose level is >140 mg/dL, or 2-hour glucose level is >120 mg/dL, drug therapy is instituted. While there is a lot of discussion on OHA versus insulin, insulin is still the gold standard therapy for management of gestational diabetes.

Summary of evidence: GOI guidelines have recommended insulin dosages based on blood sugar levels. Human Insulin premix 30:70 is preferred.

Blood glucose in mg/dL	***Insulin dose***
Between 120–160	4 units
Between 160–200	6 units
More than 200	8 units

According to the GOI guidelines, insulin doses need to be adjusted based on the levels of fasting and 2-hours postprandial blood sugar.

Blood glucose in mg/dl	***Insulin doses***
FBS normal and 2 hours PPBS is high.	Increase insulin by 2 U prebreakfast + MNT and physical exercise
If both levels are high	Insulin in two doses, same dose + 2 U prebreakfast and 4 U predinner
If PPBS is elevated	Add 2 U prebreakfast
If fasting BS is elevated	Add 2 U predinner

ACOG recommends that insulin should be the preferred therapy if glycemic control is not obtained with nonpharmacologic treatment. In the first trimester, the total daily insulin requirement is 0.7 units/kg/day, in the second trimester it is 0.8 units/kg/day, and in the third trimester, it is 0.9–1.0 units/kg/day. Dosages should be divided. Long-acting or intermediate-acting insulin in combination with short-acting insulin are given. The total daily dose of insulin is usually divided into two halves—one half is administered as basal insulin at bedtime, and the other half is divided between the three meals in the form of rapid-acting, or regular insulin before meals. Short-acting analogs (e.g., insulin lispro and aspart) are preferred over regular insulin due to more rapid onset. NPH insulin is still used but insulin glargine and detemir are available for long-acting coverage. The long-acting insulin detemir can be given in pregnancy and is reported to cause less nocturnal hypoglycemia.

Q4. What is the role of oral hypoglycemic agents in GDM?

Draft recommendation: Although insulin treatment is still the "gold standard" therapy for the regulation and control of maternal glycemic status, OHA such as glyburide and metformin can be used in gestational diabetes. They are advised when it is a challenge for pregnant women to be adherent to insulin therapy regimens because of the schedule and route of administration of Insulin.

Summary of evidence: GOI and FOGSI guidelines have provided the indications and method of usage of OHA in patients with GDM. Metformin, a biguanide, prevents gluconeogenesis in the liver resulting in an increased glucose uptake in the peripheral tissues thus normalizing the blood glucose levels.

If a patient cannot take insulin or declines, metformin can be given after counseling regarding the risks associated with metformin. Metformin can cross the placenta and there are no long-term studies on the effects of the drug in the offspring. It may be associated with preterm birth.

Starting dose: 500 mg for 1 week, increase to 500 twice daily. Baseline creatinine is estimated before initiation. Maximal dose is 2,500–3,000 mg/day in two or three divided doses.

Side effects: There may be abdominal pain and diarrhea and, hence, it is recommended to be taken with meals.

Metformin instant release and extended-release formulations work the same way to treat prediabetes and type 2 diabetes mellitus. They just differ in how quickly they are released in the body. They have similar benefits and risks, but metformin extended-release formulation tends to cause fewer side effects. Glyburide should not be used in place of insulin as studies have reported macrosomia and birth injury. The starting dose is 2.5–20 mg/day to be given in divided doses. Doses up to 30 mg may be necessary to obtain glycemic control.

Long-term outcome studies are still lacking on glyburide safety, although no short-term adverse events have been noted.

Q5. How do you monitor therapy in GDM?

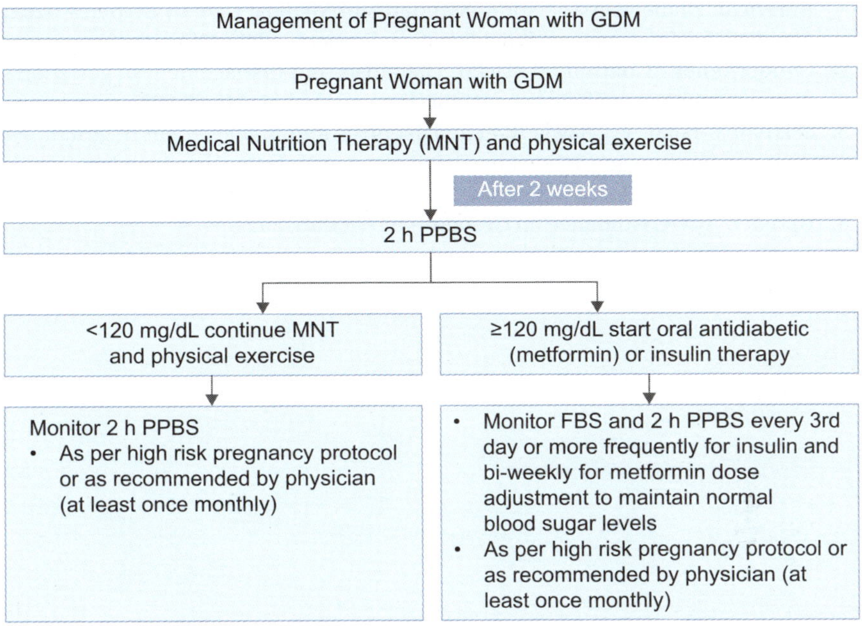

Q6. What are the indications for referral of GDM patients to higher care?

Draft recommendation: Referral of a GDM patient to a higher center is indicated only when the hospital where the patient is admitted is not fully equipped to manage the case or in apprehension of the need of specialized care for the neonate.

Summary of evidence:

- The mother is referred to a higher center based on GOI guidelines.
- When she has severe vomiting and is unable to take food orally.
- When the fasting blood sugar is >200 mg/dL with or without the use of insulin.
- When the fasting blood sugar >150 mg/dL or postbreakfast glucose level > 250 mg/dL.
- If the total dose of insulin needed for control in a day exceeds 20 units.
- If the mother develops more than one hypoglycemic episode in a day.

The neonate is referred to a higher center for the following indications:

- Two values of blood sugar <20 mg/dL despite starting 10% dextrose IV infusion
- Occurrence of convulsions
- Baby is not able to suck at repeated attempts and blood sugar is <20 mg/dL
- Failure to maintain IV line and blood sugar is <20 mg/dL.

The baby is referred to a higher center with a 10% dextrose IV infusion drip (100 mL/kg/day).

BIBLIOGRAPHY

1. American Diabetes Association. Standards of Medical Care in Diabetes—2022 Abridged for Primary Care Providers. Clin Diabetes. 2022;40(1):10-38.
2. Endocrinology Committee FOGSI. Diagnosis and management of gestational diabetes mellitus guidelines by DIPSI (Revised) Vol 17, March 2021.
3. Seshiah V, Balaji V, Chawla R, et al. Diagnosis and management of gestational diabetes mellitus guidelines by DIPSI (Revised). Int J Diab Develop Countr. 2023;43(4):485-501.
4. Updated ACOG Guidance on Gestational Diabetes, 2023.

5

CHAPTER

Medical Management of Types 1 and 2 Diabetes in Pregnancy

Ahila Ayyavoo

Q1. What are the medications to be used for diabetes in pregnancy?

Draft recommendation:

- Insulin is the ideal drug for management of diabetes in pregnancy.
- The other medications that are used in diabetes during pregnancy include oral hypoglycemic agents (OHA) such as metformin and glibenclamide. These may be more suitable for women with mild GDM.

Summary of evidence: Insulin remains the most used and best characterized drug in the management of diabetes in pregnancy across the world (Cesta et al., 2019). Insulin is the preferred drug for management of gestational diabetes mellitus (GDM), pregestational type 1 and 2 diabetes mellitus not controlled by diet, exercise, and metformin. Use of metformin has been noted to have effects similar to insulin for glycemic control and neonatal outcomes in GDM (Gui et al., 2013). No difference in pregnancy outcomes has been noted with the use of glyburide (glibenclamide) in comparison with insulin for management of GDM in some studies (Hedderson et al., 2022). But, glibenclamide is less preferred due to the risk of neonatal hypoglycemia and macrosomia (ElSayed et al., 2023). Conversion to insulin from OHA was found to be protective for perinatal mortality in the last trimester.

Q2. What is the protocol for monitoring blood sugar control?

Draft recommendation:

- Four blood sugar checks daily would help in management of GDM. One fasting blood sugar and three postprandial sugars measured 1or 2 hours after each meal would be useful in women with GDM.
- Preprandial and postprandial blood sugars for each carb meal is recommended in pregnant women with preexisting type 1 diabetes mellitus (T1DM).

Summary of evidence: The American Diabetes Association (ADA) (ElSayed et al., 2023) position statement on "Management of Diabetes in Pregnancy" recommends preprandial and postprandial monitoring of blood glucose to meet the glucose targets recommended by American College of Obstetrics and Gynecology (ACOG) ("ACOG Practice Bulletin No. 190," 2018). ACOG recommends four sugar checks daily including the initial fasting glucose and three sugars after each meal in individuals with gestational diabetes mellitus (GDM). Postprandial sugars can be measured 1 hour or 2 hours after each meal. Blood sugar checks of fewer than two times daily is usually not recommended. The frequency of blood sugar checks is more frequent in women with preexisting diabetes mellitus. These would include regular preprandial and postprandial blood sugar measurements.

Q3. What are the target levels for blood sugar control?

Draft recommendation: Blood glucose targets suggested by ACOG have been included for diagnosis of GDM with the following values on a 75 gram oral glucose tolerance test ("ACOG Practice Bulletin No. 190," 2018).

- Fasting glucose of <95 mg/dL
- 1-hour postprandial of <140 mg/dL
- 2-hour postprandial of <120 mg/dL

Summary of evidence: There is not enough supporting evidence to recommend one method of testing over another method for diagnosis of GDM (Farrar et al., 2017). These include the use of 75 g or 100 g glucose load, measuring hourly blood glucose measurement from 0 minute to 1 hour, 2 hours with or without 3 hours, one step or two steps for diagnosis, etc.

Q4. Use of glycosylated hemoglobin (HbA1c) monitoring in diabetes?

Draft recommendation:

- HbA1c of <6% without hypoglycemia is the ideal target.
- In situations where HbA1c targets of <6% could not be achieved without hypoglycemia, the target is relaxed to <7%.

The red blood cell turnover is high in pregnancy. So, HbA1c is lower during pregnancy in individuals with or without diabetes. Hence, the target HbA1c during pregnancy is lower too. The ideal goal is to have an HbA1c of <6% without hypoglycemia.(Maresh et al., 2015) HbA1c of 6–6.4% at 26 weeks of pregnancy in women with preexisting T1DM was associated with elevated risk for birth of large for gestational age. HbA1c of 6.5–6.9% was associated with preterm delivery, preeclampsia, neonatal hypoglycemia, and composite adverse outcomes. Increasing HbA1c was associated with worsening outcomes.

If an HbA1c target of <6% is difficult to achieve without hypoglycemia, the HbA1c target can be relaxed to <7% during pregnancy (ElSayed et al., 2023). But, this is secondary to measurement of regular blood sugars.

Q5. What are the different insulin regimens to be used for management of diabetes in pregnancy?

Draft recommendation:

- For women with preexisting type 1 diabetes mellitus (T1DM) or type 2 diabetes mellitus (T2DM), insulin is the preferred treatment.

- Basal bolus regimen with frequent blood sugar measurement is the ideal form of therapy in pregnant women with preexisting T1DM.
- In GDM, medical nutrition therapy, insulin and/or oral antidiabetic drugs such as metformin and glibenclamide is used. The choice of the type of insulin would be based on blood sugar values at various times of the day in GDM.

Summary of evidence: Among women with GDM, the choice of insulin regimen depends on the variations in blood glucose ("ACOG Practice Bulletin No. 190," 2018). If the lady has high blood sugars only in the fasted state in the morning, night-time administration of an intermediate insulin such as NPH or levemir or long-acting insulin such as glargine may suffice (Alfadhli, 2015). Levemir seems to have much better blood sugar profile in comparison with NPH or glargine.

If the individual has elevated blood glucose postprandially, short-acting analog insulin including insulin aspart or lispro are used just prior to the meal. This is preferred to human regular insulin as this would lower the risk of hypoglycemia.

The above recommendations are for individuals with GDM (ElSayed et al., 2023). In women with T1DM, basal bolus regimen with multiple daily dosing or insulin pump therapy is advised. Frequent blood sugar checks and dynamic insulin adjustments are necessary in pregnant women with pre-existing T1DM as they have a higher risk for hypoglycemia, ketosis, and hypoglycemia unawareness.

In women with preexisting T2DM, the insulin requirements can be huge requiring concentrated solutions as the pregnancy is a state of high insulin resistance. The dose requirement is usually around 0.7–1 unit/kg/day (Blum, 2016). The choice of insulin would be similar to GDM and would be based on blood sugar profiles.

Q6. What is the role of continuous glucose monitoring in the management?

Draft recommendation:

- Continuous glucose monitoring system (CGMS) helps in achieving preprandial and postprandial blood glucose targets to optimise "Time in Range (TIR)" in women with T1DM.
- Data is not sufficient yet for the recommendation of CGMS in GDM or T2DM in comparison to blood sugar checks with glucometer (ElSayed et al., 2023).

Summary of evidence: Several studies have proven that the TIR is superior in pregnant women with preexisting T1DM using CGMS (Feig et al., 2017). They spent less time in hypoglycemia and was associated lesser incidence of neonatal hypoglycemia, reduction in need for neonatal intensive care admissions, and lesser occurrence of large for gestational age babies.

CGMS is gaining acceptance in the management of GDM too (García-Moreno et al., 2022). It helps to improve the TIR and avoid maternal, fetal, and neonatal complications associated with GDM. But, it is yet to be formally approved.

Q7. What is the role of ketone testing in diabetes in pregnancy?

Draft recommendation:

- Ketone testing is not routinely necessary in GDM or pregnant women with preexisting T2DM.
- Ketone testing is important in pregnant women with preexisting T1DM as pregnancy is a ketosis prone state.

Summary of evidence: Presence of ketones indicate the presence of GDM or poor availability of nutrients. There is no recommendation for routine testing of ketones in GDM. It is useful to check ketones in pregnant women with preexisting T1DM during periods of other illnesses and when their blood sugars are high. Blood ketone levels of >1 mmol is considered to be hyperketonemia a level >3 mmol indicate ketoacidosis (Qian et al., 2020). This can be measured using blood ketone strips in some glucometers which have additional facility of checking ketones too.

Q8. What is the management of diabetic ketoacidosis in pregnancy (DKP)?

Draft recommendation:

- The two pillars of management of DKP are management of fluid administration and use of insulin appropriately.
- Women with DKP should be shifted to higher centers with resources including intensive care set up to manage the fluid and insulin infusion while watching for sudden acute compromise.

Summary of evidence:

- DKP is more common among women with T1DM. It is occasionally seen in women with T2DM or GDM too.
- This is precipitated by hyperemesis gravidarum, infections, starvation, insulin pump failure, and poor compliance to medications or drugs.
- The management will focus on two aspects which include appropriate intravenous (IV) fluid replacement and IV insulin therapy.
- 0.9% normal saline is first started to correct the dehydration. The fluid infusion rates will be adjusted based on the hemodynamic status. IV insulin therapy will be based on hourly blood glucose values and ketone concentrations until the patient is stable. Potassium will be added to the fluid based on the potassium concentration.

BIBLIOGRAPHY

1. ACOG Practice Bulletin No. 190: Gestational Diabetes Mellitus. Obstet Gynecol. 2018;131:e49-64.
2. Alfadhli EM. Gestational diabetes mellitus. Saudi Med J. 2015;36:399-406.
3. Blum AK. Insulin Use in Pregnancy: An Update. Diabetes. Spectr. 2016;29:92-7.
4. Cesta CE, Cohen JM, Pazzagli L, et al. Antidiabetic medication use during pregnancy: an international utilization study. BMJ Open Diabetes Res Care. 2019;7:e000759.
5. ElSayed NA, Aleppo G, Aroda VR, et al. Management of diabetes in pregnancy: standards of care in diabetes—2023. Diabetes Care. 2023;46:S254-66.
6. Farrar D, Duley L, Dowswell T, et al. Different strategies for diagnosing gestational diabetes to improve maternal and infant health. Cochrane Database Syst Rev. 2017.
7. Feig DS, Donovan LE, Corcoy R, et al. Continuous glucose monitoring in pregnant women with type 1 diabetes (CONCEPTT): a multicentre international randomised controlled trial. Lancet. 2017;390:2347-59.
8. García-Moreno RM, Benítez-Valderrama P, Barquiel B, et al. Efficacy of continuous glucose monitoring on maternal and neonatal outcomes in gestational diabetes mellitus: a systematic review and meta-analysis of randomized clinical trials. Diabet Med. 2022;39:e14703.
9. Gui J, Liu Q, Feng L. Metformin vs insulin in the management of gestational diabetes: a meta-analysis. PLoS One. 2013;8:e64585.
10. Hedderson MM, Badon SE, Pimentel N, et al. Association of glyburide and subcutaneous insulin with perinatal complications among women with gestational diabetes. JAMA Netw Open. 2022;5:e225026.
11. Maresh MJA, Holmes VA, Patterson CC, et al. Glycemic targets in the second and third trimester of pregnancy for women with Type 1 diabetes. Diabetes Care. 2015;38:34-42.
12. Mohan M, Baagar KAM, Lindow S. Management of diabetic ketoacidosis in pregnancy. Obstet Gynaecol. 2017;19:55-62.
13. Qian M, Wu N, Li L, et al. Effect of elevated ketone body on maternal and infant outcome of pregnant women with abnormal glucose metabolism during pregnancy. Diabetes Metab Syndr Obes Targets Ther. 2020;13:4581-8.

6

CHAPTER

Obstetrical Management of Hyperglycemia in Pregnancy

Uma Ram

Q1. What is the advised antenatal care in HIP?

Draft recommendation: In women with hyperglycemia in pregnancy (HIP), the adverse pregnancy outcomes are directly linked to glycemic control. Universal screening to identify women with GDM is most essential to identify the problem. Screening for comorbidities in the mother, ultrasound for identification of fetal anomalies and monitoring fetal growth, ensuring good glycemic control, and appropriate timing of delivery are the four key ingredients of antenatal care to minimize complications.

Summary of evidence: The basis for prevention of pregnancy complications is access to antenatal care with early visits in first trimester, enabling accurate dating of pregnancy. The identification of risk factors and individual planning of surveillance and possible interventions during pregnancy are helpful. Obstetrical surveillance and management include lifestyle interventions with focus on adequate gestational weight gain, balanced nutrient intake as well as physical activity are the basis of antenatal care for women with HIP.

Q2. How do we counsel women with HIP regarding antenatal care?

Draft recommendation: Women with HIP need to be counseled about their increased risk for complications. They need to be educated about glycemic targets, the need for increased antenatal visits, monitoring as well as the possibility of delivery at 38–40 weeks if they need medication for achieving glycemic control.

Summary of evidence: Lack of awareness about GDM and its impact is a major barrier to self-management. In addition, social taboos, myths as well as confused messaging on nutritional needs and exercise are some of the barriers to self-management and adherence to antenatal care (Morampudi Suman 2017). Health education among pregnant women remains a priority to resolve issues related to self-management. A recent review (N Garg 2023) suggests that mobile apps help to improve compliance to glycemic control.

Q3. How do we screen for fetal anomalies in women with HIP?

Draft recommendation: Women with pregestational diabetes and early pregnancy GDM need a good quality scan at 11–13 weeks. This needs to be performed by a trained fetal medicine specialist. Additionally, a detailed scan at 18–20 weeks with fetal ECHO is recommended.

Summary of evidence: Accurate dating is important in women with hyperglycemia as they are subjected a higher risk of undergoing labor inductions. Women exposed to hyperglycemia in early pregnancy are at increased risk of structural abnormalities. 60% of major structural abnormalities can be detected at the 11–13-week scan when performed as per protocols (ISUOG). Additionally, a detailed scan at 18–20 weeks including a detailed fetal ECHO is advised (NICE 2022).

Q4. How do we monitor fetal growth?

Draft recommendation: Fetuses of women with HIP need to have serial scans to monitor fetal growth. These should be done at 28 and 36 weeks at a minimum. In resource rich settings, 4-weekly scans can be performed from 28 weeks.

The timing of the growth scans will be influenced by presence of comorbidities and the growth trajectory of the fetus.

Summary of evidence: Evaluation of fetal growth is an important part of monitoring all pregnancies with hyperglycemia. The fetus can be affected by growth disorders depending on the level of hyperglycemia exposed to during the second and third trimester. NICE guidelines recommend 4 weekly scans from 28 weeks for women with HIP. Kjos et al. proposed that the abdominal circumference (AC) at 75th centile can be used to modify therapy in women with GDM. A meta-analysis concluded that ultrasound-guided management improves birthweight distribution, but increases the need for insulin treatment.

Q5. What is the right time to deliver?

Draft recommendation: For a pregnant woman with GDM with well-controlled sugars, induction of labor should be scheduled at or after 39 weeks pregnancy.

Poorly controlled maternal diabetes or fetal macrosomia are indications for earlier induction of labor at 38 weeks. In cases of fetal macrosomia, mothers should be informed about the risks of vaginal versus elective abdominal delivery.

The association of GDM with increased risk of stillbirth and excessive fetal growth during the latest stages of pregnancy (>38 weeks gestation) has led clinical practice to earlier induction of labor. Benefits of this approach always need to be weighed against the possibility of higher rate of cesarean section (CS), maternal infection, neonatal mortality, and morbidity. GDM by itself is not an indication for CS and mode of delivery should be a shared decision between clinician and mother. Specific conditions such as macrosomia, fetal distress, and risk of intrauterine death are factors leading to abdominal delivery.

Summary of evidence: Observational studies have shown that elective induction before 38 weeks does not necessarily reduce the risk of macrosomia or shoulder dystocia. However, some of them were underpowered and additionally did not address stillbirth risk.

A recent meta-analysis suggests that induction reduces macrosomia and perineal trauma but did not impact CS rates and perinatal or neonatal morbidity. The overall quality of studies was stated as low to very low with only three RCTs, one of which was nearly 30 years ago. There is global consensus that the mode and timing of delivery should be individualized and based on maternal or fetal complications.

Research gaps: There is very little good quality evidence to guide timing of delivery in GDM. As there are ethnic differences both in fetal growth and stillbirth risks, there is an urgent need for studies in this area from our country.

Q6. How do we prevent stillbirth?

Draft recommendation: Screening and identification of HIP is the key first step in reduction of stillbirth. Ensuring good glycemic control with appropriate and frequent monitoring of sugars is recommended. Monitoring fetal growth is important to identify SGA and LGA fetuses who are at increased risk of stillbirth. The LGA fetuses and poor glycemic control appear to be the higher risk subgroup among women with HIP.

Summary of evidence: Stillbirth in women with HIP is often the result of a metabolic change caused by hyperglycemia in the fetus that induces acidosis and hypoxia. Since it is a metabolic problem, tests of placental function such as Doppler and CTG are not effective tools though they are used for surveillance. However, other comorbidities such as higher BMI and preeclampsia can contribute to stillbirth.

The risk of SB in women with GDM varies with the method of diagnosis, glycemic control, maternal comorbidities, and ethnicity. This could be the reason for conflicting data on the impact of management on stillbirth in GDM. The risk of SB is also impacted by gestational age and increases to exceed the risk of expectant management at 39 weeks.

Stillbirth risk is also impacted by fetal size and growth with the LGA fetuses being more at risk. The key to prevention of stillbirth is identification of hyperglycemia. Studies have shown that women who are not screened have higher stillbirth rates when compared to women who are screened. Good glycemic control is most important since it reduces fetal hyperglycemia and the subsequent metabolic changes.

Q7. When is it appropriate to perform a cesarean?

Draft recommendation: Cesarean section should be offered and discussed with women who have large for gestational (LGA) fetuses which are above the 95th centile for growth because of the higher chance of birth trauma and emergency cesarean section. The pros and cons of an elective induction of labor need to be discussed. It is important that the elective section is not performed before 38 completed weeks due to the risk of respiratory problems in the neonate.

Summary of evidence: Diabetes, by itself, is not an indication for cesarean delivery, in the absence of any other obstetric indication. Fetal macrosomia could be an indication for cesarean birth due to the risk of shoulder dystocia.

The ACOG recommends prophylactic cesarean birth to prevent brachial plexus injury when the EFW is >4,500 g in women with diabetes, even though the ultrasound prediction of macrosomia is imprecise.

Research gaps: There is a need for data from India to determine what is the EFW above which the risk of birth injury is high to offer elective cesarean section.

Q8. How do we manage labor in a woman with HIP?

Draft recommendation: Multidisciplinary perinatal care is paramount for all women with HIP. A written policy/guideline, agreed upon by a multidisciplinary diabetes care team, is very important, especially in pregestational diabetics. This helps to ensure that a standard care is given by all the intrapartum care providers. It is prudent to monitor labor in women with HIP electronically.

Summary of evidence: The use of a partograph or labor care guide is very important in monitoring labor in women with HIP for early recognition of slow progress. A risk score that was developed to predict the risk of cesarean in women with gestational diabetes found that nulliparity, insulin use, and excessive gestational weight gain were significant predictors of both elective and emergency cesarean delivery.

Oral hypoglycemics are stopped with the onset of active labor. Periodic assessment of capillary blood glucose is advised to ensure that the values are in range, and covered with insulin if needed.

Insulin administration is switched to sliding scale/variable rate intravenous insulin infusion (VRIII) in active labor. Management of hyperglycemia in labor should be done with the help of an endocrinologist who is involved in the care of the woman.

BIBLIOGRAPHY

1. Alberico S, Erenbourg A, Hod M, et al.; GINEXMAL Group. Immediate delivery or expectant management in gestational diabetes at term: the GINEXMAL randomised controlled trial. BJOG. 2017;124(4):669-77.
2. Balsells M, García-Patterson A, Gich I, et al. Ultrasound-guided compared to conventional treatment in gestational diabetes leads to improved birthweight but more insulin treatment: systematic review and meta-analysis. Acta Obstet Gynecol Scand. 2014;93:144-51.

3. Brown J, Ceysens G, Boulvain M. Exercise for pregnant women with gestational diabetes for improving maternal and fetal outcomes. Cochrane Database Syst Rev. 2017;6(6):CD012202.
4. Cooray SD, Boyle JA, Soldatos G, et al. Development, validation and clinical utility of a risk prediction model for adverse pregnancy outcomes in women with gestational diabetes: The PeRSonal GDM model. EClinicalMedicine. 2022;52:101637.
5. Garg N, Arunan SK, Arora S, et al. Application of mobile technology for disease and treatment monitoring of gestational diabetes mellitus among pregnant women: a systematic review. J Diab Sci Technol. 2022;16(2):491-7.
6. Hannah W, Bhavadharini B, Beks H, et al. Global burden of early pregnancy gestational diabetes mellitus (eGDM): a systematic review. Acta Diabetol. 2022;59:403-27.
7. Hinkle SN, Buck Louis GM, Rawal S, et al. A longitudinal study of depression and gestational diabetes in pregnancy and the postpartum period. Diabetologia. 2016;59:2594-602.
8. Hivert MF, Backman H, Benhalima K, et al. Pathophysiology from preconception, during pregnancy, and beyond. Lancet. 2024;404(10448):158-74.
9. Hod M, Kapur A, Sacks DA, et al. The International Federation of Gynecology and Obstetrics (FIGO) Initiative on gestational diabetes mellitus: a pragmatic guide for diagnosis, management, and care. Int J Gynaecol Obstet. 2015;131(Suppl 3):S173-211.
10. Kjos SL, Schaefer-Graf U, Sardesi S, et al. A randomized controlled trial utilizing glycemic plus fetal ultrasound parameters vs glycemic parameters to determine insulin therapy in gestational diabetes with fasting hyperglycemia. Diabetes Care. 2001;24:1904-10.
11. Luo R, Wen W, Corsi DJ, et al. Comparison of adverse maternal and perinatal outcomes between induction and expectant management among women with gestational diabetes mellitus at term pregnancy: a systematic review and meta-analysis. BMC Pregnancy Childbirth. 2023;23:509.
12. McElwee ER, Oliver EA, McFarling K, et al. Risk of stillbirth in pregnancies complicated by diabetes, stratified by fetal growth. Obstet Gynecol. 2023;141(4):801-9.
13. National Guidelines for Diagnosis & Management of Gestational Diabetes Mellitus, 2014.
14. Phaloprakarn C, Tangjitgamol S. Risk score for predicting primary cesarean delivery in women with gestational diabetes mellitus. BMC Pregnancy Childbirth. 2020;20:607.
15. Rosenstein MG, Cheng YW, Snowden JM, et al. The risk of stillbirth and infant death stratified by gestational age in women with gestational diabetes. Am J Obstet Gynecol. 2012;206(4):309.e1-7.
16. Sanabria-Martínez G, García-Hermoso A, Poyatos-León R, et al. Effectiveness of physical activity interventions on preventing gestational diabetes mellitus and excessive maternal weight gain: a meta-analysis. BJOG. 2015;122(9):1167-74.
17. Suman M, Gayathri B, Arun G, et al. The challenges and recommendations for gestational diabetes mellitus care in India: a review. Front Endocrinol. 2017;8:56.
18. Sweeting A, Hannah W, Backman H, et al. Epidemiology and management of gestational diabetes. Lancet. 2024;404(10448):175-92.
19. Ye W, Luo C, Huang J, et al. Gestational diabetes mellitus and adverse pregnancy outcomes: systematic review and meta-analysis. BMJ. 2022;377:e067946.

CHAPTER 7

Neonatal Perspectives in the Management of Gestational Diabetes Mellitus

S Karthikeyan

Q1. What is the delivery room management of neonate born to gestational diabetes mellitus (GDM) mother?

Draft recommendation: The need for neonatal resuscitation should be made based on gestational age, predicted birthweight, prenatally diagnosed congenital anomalies, mode of delivery, and any complications during labor.

Summary of evidence: *Cloherty's South Asian Textbook of Pediatrics* suggests that the following needs to be done for a neonate born to a mother with HIP:

- Anticipate increased risk of need for resuscitation at birth.
- Examine the baby for bruises, hematoma on scalp, brachial plexus injury, paucity of limb movements because of the higher risk of macrosomia.
- Do a pulse oximetry evaluation as the infants have a risk of respiratory distress syndrome (RDS), and congenital heart disease.

Q2. What are the indications for care in NICU?

Draft recommendation: It is not necessary to admit all babies born to mothers with HIP. Admission is needed if there are complications.

Summary of evidence: *Cloherty's South Asian Textbook of Pediatrics* suggests that admission is needed in following indications:

- Preterm birth
- Fetal growth restriction
- Large baby of >4 kg weight
- RDS, transient tachypnea of the newborn (TTN)
- Abnormal pulse oximetry screening
- Hypoglycemia, hypocalcemia, and polycythemia

Q3. What are the basic tests to be done in GDM baby in postnatal ward?

Draft recommendation: ICMR guidelines suggest that capillary blood glucose monitoring be done at 2, 6, 12, 24, 48, and 72 hours of life. The tests that are recommended to monitor the baby include blood glucose, serum calcium, and hematocrit to look for polycythemia.

Summary of evidence: *Cloherty's South Asian Textbook of Pediatrics* suggests that serum calcium levels and hematocrit should be done only if the baby is lethargic, and has respiratory distress or seizures.

Q4. What are the challenges in managing hypoglycemia in GDM baby?

Draft recommendation: Asymptomatic hypoglycemia is common in babies born to mothers with HIP. Serial blood glucose measurement is needed in these babies.

Summary of evidence: ICMR guidelines suggest that serial blood glucose measurements are needed. The neonates should not be fed 5%,10%, or 25% dextrose as a substitute for breast milk. The mother should be supported for early initiation and regular breastfeeding.

Q5. What is the management of neonatal hypoglycemia?

Draft recommendation:

- Blood glucose <45 mg/dL should be considered as hypoglycemia.
- Symptoms and signs such as lethargy, jitteriness, convulsions, tremors, apnea or tachypnea, weak cry, and difficulty in feeding should be looked for.
- If there are no symptoms but the blood sugar levels are low, it is treated as asymptomatic hypoglycemia.

Summary of evidence: ICMR guidelines have suggested a stepwise management for neonatal hypoglycemia.

ASYMPTOMATIC

- Immediate supervised feeding
- Breastfeeding or a measured volume of expressed breast milk (formula milk if EBM not available) by paladai or gavage

RE-CHECK BG AFTER 1 HOUR

If BG ≥45 mg/dL
- Continue feeds
- Continue BG monitoring every 6 hourly for 24 hours

Start IV glucose infusion if:
BG <45 despite one attempt of feeding
OR
Baby becomes symptomatic

PREVENTION OF HYPOGLYCEMIA

- Support mother for early initiation and regular breastfeeding
- Maintain normothermia
- Do not feed 5%, 10% or 25% dextrose as a substitute for breast milk

PRACTICAL POINTS

- Avoid >12.5–15% dextrose infusion through a peripheral vein
- Use a syringe/infusion pump to deliver glucose
- Avoid frequent dextrose boluses
- Send blood in fluoride or oxalate vial for laboratory glucose estimation
- Always search for an underlying cause – polycythemia, sepsis, meningitis, hypothermia, IUGR
- Do not give antibiotics unless sepsis is suspected (refer to STW on sepsis)

SYMPTOMATIC OR BG <20 mg/dL

- IV bolus: 2 mL/kg 10% dextrose
- Start IV infusion of dextrose at a glucose infusion rate (GIR) of 6 mg/kg/min

Re-check BG every 30 minutes till 2 values ≥45 mg/dL and then every 6 hours

BG <45 mg/dL

Increase GIR @ 2 mg/kg/min till max GIR 12 mg/kg/min

Refractory hypoglycemia: High (>12 mg/kg/min for 24 hours) or persistent (>7 days) GIR requirement

CONSIDER DRUGS* AND REFER TO HIGHER CENTRE

BG ≥45 mg/dL

Euglycemic for 24 hours on IV fluids

- Wean @ 2 mg/kg/min every 6 hourly
- Increase oral feeds
- Monitor BG every 6 hourly

Stop IV fluids when euglycemic on GIR 4 mg/kg/min

***DRUGS FOR REFRACTORY HYPOGLYCEMIA**

- Hydrocortisone: 5 mg/kg/day IV in two divided doses
- Diazoxide: 10–25 mg/kg/day PO in three divided doses
- Glucagon: 300 µg/kg SC or IM
- Octreotide: 2–10 µg/kg/day SC

Q6. What is the long-term follow-up for GDM baby?

Draft recommendation: Infants born to mothers with HIP are more prone for metabolic syndrome, obesity, diabetes, and impaired neurodevelopmental outcome. They should be regularly monitored for BMI, development of high blood pressure, altered lipid profiles, and increased blood glucose levels.

Summary of evidence: *Cloherty's South Asian Textbook of Pediatrics* suggests that maternal diabetes and prenatal exposure to hypoglycemia have been shown to increase long-term metabolic and neurodevelopmental problems in the offspring.

Q7. What are the effects of maternal therapy with insulin and OHA on the glycemic status of the neonate?

Draft recommendation: Insulin therapy results in newborn normoglycemia and reduces risk of the risk of macrosomia.

Summary of evidence: There is no evidence on the neonatal effects of maternal pharmacologic therapy.

Research gaps: Studies are needed on the effects of maternal pharmacological therapy on the newborn.

Q8. What are the glycemic effects in the fetus in each trimester?

Draft recommendation:
- Congenital anomalies are more common in mothers with pregestational diabetes than in mothers with gestational diabetes mellitus.
- The chances of developing diabetic embryopathy is more common in the first trimester if mothers have uncontrolled hyperglycemia.

Summary of evidence: Congenital malformations are two- to fourfold higher in pregestational diabetes. Congenital malformations and diabetic embryopathy are common in mothers who have uncontrolled blood sugars in the first trimester. They are not common in mothers who develop GDM in the late trimesters of pregnancy. Neonates of mothers who have uncontrolled blood sugars in the second and third trimester have a higher chance of developing macrosomia, hyperinsulinemia which can cause impaired lung maturation leading onto respiratory distress, and polycythemia because of increased erythropoietin.

BIBLIOGRAPHY

1. Behboudi-Gandevani S, Bidhendi-Yarandi R, Panahi MH, et al. The effect of mild gestational diabetes mellitus treatment on adverse pregnancy outcomes: a systemic review and meta-analysis. Front Endocrinal. 2021;12:640004.

2. Eichenwald EC, Hansen AR, Martin CR, et al. Cloherty and Stark's Manual of Neonatal care second South Asian edition. Gurugram, Haryana (India): Wolters Kluwer (India) Pvt. Ltd.; 2023.
3. Standard Treatment Workflow (STW). Neonatal Hypoglycemia ICD-10-P70.4 stw.icmr.org.in.
4. Subiabre M, Silva L, Toledo F, et al. Insulin therapy and its consequences for the mother, foetus, and newborn in gestational diabetes mellitus. Biochimica et Biophysica Acta (BBA) - Molecular Basis of Disease. 1864(9):Part B,Pages 2949-2956.

8

CHAPTER

Postpartum Management (Short-term and Long-term Care) in Hyperglycemia in Pregnancy

Veerasamy Seshiah, Bhavatharini Aruyerchelvan, R Aruyerchelvan

SHORT-TERM CARE

Q1. What is the management of a patient with HIP in the postpartum period?

Draft recommendation: Women with HIP should get routine postpartum care. Wound care is mandatory as there is a higher rate of infection. Exclusive breastfeeding is advocated and should be continued as long as possible. This is important to avoid neonatal hypoglycemia and for the long-term health of the mother (FIGO).

If the mother had GDM and had been advised insulin or OHA during pregnancy, she can discontinue the medications in the immediate postpartum period. The blood sugars should be checked at least once in the hospital. In women with insulin-treated preexisting diabetes, the doses of insulin are reduced immediately after the birth of the baby.

There is a higher risk of postpartum depression in HIP (NICE).

Summary of evidence: Women with HIP have a slightly higher rate of postpartum infection. FIGO advocates measures to identify early signs of genitourinary, uterine, and surgical site infections (episiotomy and cesarean delivery). It is mandatory if the delivery is prolonged or there was a need for operative intervention.

For GDM women, insulin or oral hypoglycemics can be discontinued immediately postdelivery if blood sugar is within normal limits (ACOG, 2018). According to ADA, the insulin resistance decreases rapidly after delivery in women who had type 2 diabetes (T2D) during pregnancy. The insulin requirements are half the dose requirements of the prepregnancy period in the first few days of the postpartum period. The blood glucose levels are monitored to identify the correct dose needed. They are at a higher risk of developing hypoglycemia in the postpartum period and should be encouraged to have a meal or snack before or after insulin injections.

Breastfeeding reduces the risk of development of T2D in women with GDM (Ley SH, 2020 and Stuebe AM, 2005). According to the American Diabetic Association (ADA), breast feeding can increase the occurrence of overnight hypoglycemia in women with diabetes and insulin dosing may need to be adjusted. Postpartum depression is more common among patients with diabetes (preexisting or gestational) than in postpartum patients without diabetes and they should be screened for the disease (Kozhimannil, 2009).

Q2. What are the medications to be continued in the postpartum period in diabetes in HIP?

Draft recommendation: Most women with GDM will not need medication in the postpartum period. However, preexisting diabetics and overt diabetics who were identified only in the pregnancy may need medication to achieve glycemic control. Insulin can be used safely when needed for achieving glycemic control. Metformin and glyburide are safe to use in the postpartum period.

Summary of evidence: Preexisting diabetic women need major insulin changes postpartum. The American Diabetes Association (ADA, 2021) advises lowering insulin doses by 30–50% shortly after delivery. This lowering is needed because insulin resistance drops rapidly after placental delivery (Blumer et al., 2013). Due to limited transfer into breast milk, metformin and glyburide are breastfeeding-friendly (Hale & Rowe, 2017). Women can restart metformin and glyburide postpartum without risking breastfeeding infants, according to the ADA (2021).

Q3. How should her glycemic status be monitored in the postpartum period?

Draft recommendation: A fasting blood sugar (FBS) and a 2-hour postprandial blood sugar (PPBS) are done on the third postpartum day. At 6 weeks postpartum, a 75-g glucose tolerance test (GTT) is done (GOI).

Summary of evidence: The levels to monitor glycemic status in the postpartum period is as per GOI guidelines. The normal values are as follows:

- Fasting plasma glucose: ≥126 mg/dL
- 75 g OGTT 2-hour blood glucose
- Normal: <140 mg/dL
- Impaired glucose tolerance (IGT): 140–199 mg/dL
- Diabetes: ≥200 mg/dL

Test report	*Recommendation*
Normal	Counseled about lifestyle modifications like control of weight and physical exercise
Positive	Advised to consult a physician

LONG-TERM CARE

Q1. What are the screening strategies for providing long-term care in women with HIP?

Draft recommendation: A 75-g OGTT at 6–12 weeks in the fasting state is done in the postpartum period and they need to be screened for their risk of cardiovascular diseases (CVD) and metabolic syndrome on a regular basis in the long term.

Summary of evidence: The ADA (2021) has suggested that for women with a history of GDM, a 75-g OGTT should be done at about 4–12 weeks postpartum. According to ADA, OGTT is used in the postpartum period for detecting glucose intolerance. It is more sensitive than glycosylated hemoglobin (HbA1C).

According to the ADA (2021), screening should be performed for life or at shorter intervals if risk factors are present. Annual screening with physical examinations is useful in estimating cardiovascular disease risk factors, cancer detection, and to reinforce lifestyle changes and promote weight control, which prevent type 2 diabetes. Identifying persistent glucose intolerance early allows for effective intervention and management (Ratner et al., 2008). Due to higher rates of T2DM, CVD and other negative consequences, GDM women should be monitored for a lifetime (Bellamy et al., 2009).

Women with GDM have a high probability of developing CVD in later life (Kramer et al., 2019). ACOG (2018) advises these women to have regular cardiovascular risk assessments, including BMI, waist to hip ratio, and lipid profile. Long-term care should include screening for metabolic syndrome components. According to Lauenborg et al. (2005), 40% of GDM women had metabolic syndrome 9.8 years postpartum, compared to 5.5% of controls.

Gaps in research: The potential of using an alternative to an OGTT such as an HbA1c needs to be studied to help to improve the acceptance of postpartum screening.

Q2. What is the advice regarding lifestyle changes in a mother with HIP?

Draft recommendations: All women with HIP need to be given advice about lifestyle. This includes recommendation on diet, exercise, and postpartum weight loss. Dietary recommendation should include higher fiber consumption, reduced carbohydrate and refined sugars, and increased plant-based protein.

Summary of evidence: Women with GDM have a higher risk of developing T2DM later in life. They should be counseled for lifestyle management on diet and exercise. These are important for reducing noncommunicable diseases (NCD) in the future (GOI).

There should be an interdisciplinary management of mothers with GDM in the long-term care.

The follow-up can be linked to the child's vaccination and health check-up (FIGO). Women who had GDM with evidence of prediabetes in pregnancy should be advised to follow intensive lifestyle management and metformin to reduce the development of diabetes in the future (ADA).

Diet recommendations: According to ADA (2021), the recommended diet includes whole grains, fruits, vegetables, lean sources of proteins, and healthy fats. A Mediterranean-style diet lowered T2DM risk by 40% in GDM women (Tobias et al., 2014).

Exercise recommendations: Women with HIP should exercise regularly to prevent T2DM and improve their health. According to the ADA (2021), individuals must do 150 minutes of aerobic activity per week, twice-weekly resistance training, and short bouts of physical activity to break up prolonged sitting as sitting is modern smoking. Bao et al. (2014) observed that GDM women who exercised 150 minutes per week had a 47% lower incidence of T2DM than inactive women.

Strategies for weight management:

- Establish realistic weight loss goals (5–7% of baseline weight for overweight or obese women).
- Regarding weight, Ehrlich et al. (2011) observed that woman who has prepregnancy weight within 1 year of childbirth was at a lesser risk for developing type 2 than woman with retained weight.
- Women with GDM should follow lifelong screening for T2DM or prediabetes at least once in 3 years.
- Women with GDM should have preconceptional screening for T2DM and preconceptional care to treat hyperglycemia and prevent congenital anomalies. Self-care support and psychosocial assessment should be included for long-term care.

Q3. How can the intergenerational transmission of noncommunicable diseases be prevented?

Draft recommendation: Intergenerational transfer is best prevented by planning pregnancies, identifying risk factors and optimizing maternal health prior to pregnancy. Once hyperglycemia is identified in a pregnancy, we can reduce the intergenerational impact by tight glycemic control throughout pregnancy, breastfeeding promotion. Subsequently, the newborn will benefit from early-life nutrition and physical activity interventions and regular monitoring of offspring growth and development.

Summary of evidence: According to the ADA (2021), all women of reproductive age with diabetes should have preconception counseling at the earliest, and ideally, from adolescence.

- Highlighting glycemic control before and throughout pregnancy
- Addressing weight, food, and exercise risk factors
- Pregnancy medication safety review
- Screening for diabetic complications
- Folic acid supplementation

Since fertility comes back within 6 weeks after birth, counseling with a woman and her partner on contraception is a primary way of preventing pregnancy with uncontrolled type 2 diabetes mellitus, at the same time optimizing weight, lifestyle, and interval before the subsequent pregnancy (Alexopoulos A, et al. 2019). Interpregnancy intervals shorter than 1 year are linked with gestational diabetes and postnatal weight gain. The WHO currently proposes an interpregnancy interval of at least 24 months for all women (Black KT, et al. 2022).

Research gaps: Studies are needed to understand the links between maternal health and NCDs.

Future research: Tests for glycemic status and metabolic diseases should be cost-effective and simple so that adherence will not be a problem.

BIBLIOGRAPHY

1. Alexopoulos AS, Blair R, Peters AL. Management of preexisting diabetes in pregnancy: a review. JAMA. 2019;321(18):1811-9.
2. American Diabetes Association (2020). Management of diabetes in pregnancy: standards of medical care in diabetes—2020. Diabetes care. 2020;43(Suppl 1):S183-92.
3. Boushra M, Rahman O. Postpartum Infection. 2023. In: StatPearls [Internet]. Treasure Island (FL): StatPearls Publishing; 2024.
4. Hod M, Kapur A, Sacks DA, et al. The International Federation of Gynecology and Obstetrics (FIGO) Initiative on gestational diabetes mellitus: a pragmatic guide for diagnosis, management, and care. Int J Gynaecol Obstet. 2015;131(Suppl 3):S173-211.
5. Kozhimannil KB, Pereira MA, Harlow BL. Association between diabetes and perinatal depression among low-income mothers. JAMA. 2009;301(8):842-7.
6. Ley SH, Chavarro JE, Li M, et al. Lactation duration and long-term risk for incident Type 2 diabetes in women with a history of gestational diabetes mellitus. Diabetes Care. 2020;43(4):793-8.
7. Platts J, Agarwal N. Updated NICE guidelines for diabetes and pregnancy: new challenges for primary care. Diabetes Primary Care. 2015;17:88-92.
8. Stuebe AM, Rich-Edwards JW, Willett WC, et al. Duration of lactation and incidence of type 2 diabetes. JAMA. 2005;294(20):2601-10.

CHAPTER 9

Contraceptive Choices in Hyperglycemia in Pregnancy

AG Radhika, Archana Chaudhary

Q1. What are the contraceptive choices in women with hyperglycemia in pregnancy?

Draft recommendation:

- Due to the effectiveness, acceptability, and tolerance, combined oral contraceptions (COCs) are the method of choice for women with deranged blood sugars.
- During the first 21 days following delivery of women with GDM or diabetes mellitus, all combined hormonal contraceptives are contraindicated due to increased risk for thrombotic events.
- After 42 days postpartum, all nonbreastfeeding women can use COC regardless of pregnancy-related thromboembolic risk factors. However, if the woman is breastfeeding, COCs are best avoided till 6 months postpartum.
- COCs should be avoided in diabetic postpartum women with cardiovascular and microvascular complications namely retinopathy (ischemic or proliferative), active macular edema, or nephropathy with persistent proteinuria and diabetes for >20 years.
- *Nonoral combined contraception:* Contraindications and precautions for diabetic women are the same as those for combined oral contraceptives.
- Progestin only pills and implants can be started anytime in breastfeeding women with GDM and in women with diabetes mellitus with or without complications.
- Newer generation of progestins such as gestodene, dienogest, drospirenone, and nomegestrol-acetate containing combined hormonal contraceptives are safe for use in women with hyperglycemia without cardiovascular and microvascular complications 6 months after delivery in breastfeeding women and 6 weeks after delivery if she is not breastfeeding.
- Progestin only pill containing newer progestin desogestrel is safe in breastfeeding postpartum female with hyperglycemia without complications. It can be started immediately after delivery in nonbreastfeeding female.
- Progestin only pills can also be used in diabetes mellitus with cardiovascular and microvascular complications (WHO MEC-2).

- Injectable progesterone for contraception is preferably avoided in women with history of gestational diabetes.
- Women with GDM/DM can also safely opt for intrauterine contraceptive device.
- Women with DM can use any emergency contraception.
- IUCD/LNG-IUS can be chosen as a postpartum contraceptive in well-selected cases with no evidence of sepsis, inserted within 48 hours of delivery in GDM and diabetes mellitus.
- Female sterilization is also an option after delivery in women with GDM and diabetes mellitus.
- *Contraindications* to combined oral contraceptives:
  - Dyslipidemia and hypertriglyceridemia
  - High blood pressure
  - Smokers
  - Nephropathy
  - Proliferating retinopathy, and
  - Diabetes with a progression of >20 years
- Following are *not a contraindication* to use of COCs.
  - Simple retinopathy
  - Microalbuminuria
  - Poor control of diabetes

Summary of evidence: Factors that influence the choice of contraception include age, diabetes type, cardiovascular risk factors, psychosocial context, and risk of sexually transmitted diseases. Hormonal contraceptives have no significant effect on *carbohydrate metabolism* in healthy women or those who are overweight and at risk for diabetes. However, women with vasculopathy and those with long-standing DM for more than 20 years should avoid using COCs. There is little change in the metabolism of glucose in diabetics who take progesterone only contraception. Among at-risk women (obese or with a history of gestational diabetes), injectable progestin-only contraception is associated with fasting blood sugar elevation, insulin resistance, and increased diabetes risk. It is contraindicated in diabetics. In diabetic and in older women, IUDs are the method of choice.

Centchroman as contraception following HIP:

Draft recommendations: Centchroman, a nonsteroidal selective estrogen receptor modulator, is safe for use by women with hyperglycemia in pregnancy as a contraceptive.

Evidence and justification: Centchroman has no adverse effect on cholesterol, triglycerides, and HDL cholesterol or blood sugars, and is considered safe in women with GDM or preexisting DM.

Evidence gap: Research on contraception in women with hyperglycemia during pregnancy such as gestational diabetes mellitus (GDM) reveals several evidence gaps including:

- *Long-term health outcomes:* There is a lack of data on the long-term health outcomes associated with the use of various contraceptive methods in women with a history of GDM.
- *Safety and metabolic effects:* The metabolic safety of hormonal contraception, particularly combined oral contraceptives, in women with a history of GDM or persistent glucose intolerance needs further study.
- *Contraceptive efficacy and adherence:* There are gaps in understanding the efficacy and adherence patterns of different contraceptive methods in women with previous hyperglycemia in pregnancy.
- *Behavioral and psychosocial factors:* Research into how behavioral and psychosocial factors affect contraceptive choices in this population is lacking.
- *Prepregnancy planning and education:* Evidence on the effectiveness of prepregnancy education and counseling specifically tailored to women with a history of GDM is insufficient.

BIBLIOGRAPHY

1. ACOG. Practice Bulletin no. 2019;206.
2. FSRH Guideline on Contraception after Pregnancy, 2017.
3. MOHFW—FP Revised guidelines, 2021.
4. NICE guideline, 2020.
5. WHO MEC wheel, 2022.
6. WHO Medical Eligibility Criteria for Contraceptive use, 2015.

10

CHAPTER

Complications of Hyperglycemia in Pregnancy

Charmila Ayyavoo

Q1. What are the maternal complications of GDM?

Draft recommendation: There is a higher chance of developing hypertensive disorders of pregnancy which includes pre-eclampsia, birth trauma, polyhydramnios, and higher incidence of caesarean deliveries in the mother. The mother has a risk of developing type 2 diabetes later in her life.

Summary of evidence: FIGO, NICE, and GOI guidelines have emphasized optimum glucose control of the mother to prevent the complications in the mother.

Research gap: The levels of glucose control which prevent maternal complications have not been elucidated yet. Glycosylated hemoglobin cannot be used to identify blood glucose control during pregnancy. Other tests are needed to assess blood glucose control.

Q2. What are the fetal complications of GDM?

Draft recommendation: There is a higher chance of perinatal and neonatal morbidities in babies born to mothers with HIP. The complications in the fetus include big baby, shoulder dystocia during labor, and birth injuries. The baby can also develop long-term complications like a higher chance of obesity, dysregulated carbohydrate metabolism, and diabetes as adults.

Summary of evidence: The guidelines by FIGO, GOI, and NICE have dealt about the short-term and long-term complications in babies born to mothers with HIP.

Research gaps: Intrauterine death is a common cause of perinatal mortality in women with HIP especially in diabetic pregnancies. There are no sensitive tests available to predict the occurrence of intrauterine compromise.

Q3. What are the maternal and fetal complications in diabetic pregnancies?

Draft recommendation: There is a higher chance of developing maternal and fetal complications in diabetic pregnancies due to the higher levels of blood sugar. The mother can suffer spontaneous miscarriages, pre-eclampsia, congenital anomalies, macrosomia, prolonged labor, obstructed labor, atonicity of uterus, intrauterine death, stillbirth, postpartum hemorrhage, and infections.

The baby can suffer from neonatal hyperglycemia, electrolyte abnormalities, hyperbilirubinemia, and respiratory distress of the newborn.

There is also a higher chance of the baby developing obesity, hypertension, and type 2 diabetes later in life.

Summary of evidence: ADA has enumerated the maternal and fetal complications of mothers with pregestational diabetes.

Q4. What are the co-morbidities which can worsen in a woman with diabetes and pregnancy?

Draft recommendation: There is a high risk for developing hypertension in diabetic pregnancies. It is high in both type 1 and 2 diabetic pregnancies. Pregnancy losses are more common in first trimester in type 1 diabetes and more common in third trimester in type 2 diabetes.

Women with type 1 or type 2 can develop retinopathy. Maintaining women with retinopathy in an euglycemic state is very important to prevent worsening of the condition during pregnancy.

Summary of evidence: Women with diabetes in pregnancy should be given 60–150 mg (usual dose of 81 mg/day) to reduce the risk of development of preeclampsia. According to ADA, blood pressure of 135/85 mm Hg is treated for promotion of long-term maternal health. Blood pressure is maintained at 120/80 mm Hg for the well-being of the baby.

ACE inhibitors, angiotensin receptor blockers, statins are stopped in the preconceptional period of diabetic mothers to prevent teratogenicity.

The rapid control of blood glucose levels in mothers with retinopathy can cause worsening. The blood sugars should be brought under control gradually. According to NICE guidelines, the mother is offered screening for retinopathy in the first antenatal visit, at 16–20 weeks, and at 28 weeks of pregnancy. If she has a high HbA1c in the first trimester with retinopathy, rapid control of sugars can be attempted to prevent worsening of retinopathy according to NICE guidelines. Diabetic retinopathy is not a contraindication for a vaginal birth.

Q5. What is the management of diabetic ketoacidosis?

Draft recommendation: Women with type 1 diabetes mellitus are prone for development of diabetic ketoacidosis (DKA). Patients with type 2 diabetes are also prone but to a lesser extent.

Diabetes patients are given ketone strips and counseled on the risks for DKA development and management.

If a mother is unwell, she should be screened for DKA.

Summary of evidence: The ADA has given recommendations on DKA in pregnancy. Pregnancy is a ketogenic state and women develop DKA at lower levels than in the nonpregnant state.

According to NICE guidelines, if a diabetic mother complains of tiredness, she should be checked for DKA. She is admitted for higher care. DKA in pregnancy is associated with a higher risk of stillbirth. If a mother develops DKA, she will need 10% dextrose intravenously to meet the demands of the placenta and the baby in the third trimester.

The management of DKA in pregnancy should be by a multi-disciplinary team.

Q6. How can fetal death be prevented in HIP?

Draft recommendation: Intrauterine fetal death can happen unexpectedly in diabetic pregnancies. Conventional fetal testing is not very sensitive in predicting fetal death.

Summary of evidence: According to NICE guidelines, usage of fetal well-being tests like Doppler studies of the fetal umbilical artery, nonstress tests, and other biophysical tests cannot predict intrauterine fetal death.

Research gap: New tests like amniotic fluid erythropoietin levels and MRI spectroscopy have been studied for predicting fetal death but they there is no clinical evidence of effectiveness yet.